Consultations & Appointments

Form Organiser

For Reflexologists

(Revised)

by Galina St George

Therapist name..

Address...

....

Telephone number...

REFLEXOLOGY CONSULTATION FORM

Therapist/ Clinic	Address, tel. number	Date
Client's Name	Gender	Doctor's name
Client's address	Age	Doctor's address
Tel. number	Occupation	Doctor's tel. number

GENERAL HEALTH

Symptoms presented by the client for treatment (if any)	General Health

LIFESTYLE/ BACKGROUND INFORMATION

Occupation	Stress level (1-10):	Diet:	Eating patterns
Family circumstances	Exercise	Fluid intake	Sleeping patterns
Relaxation	Alcohol intake	Smoker/non-smoker	Bowels

MEDICAL HISTORY

PAST MEDICAL HISTORY	PRESENT HEALTH
Recent operations	Medical conditions
Serious illnesses, accidents, injuries	Medication taken
Past treatments (received from other therapists or medical ones). When and why?	Current treatments

CONTRA-INDICATIONS/ CAUTIONS

Diabetes/Epilepsy	Arthritis / Rheumatism	Back / Neck Problems
Contagious/Infectious diseases	Moles (large, irregular), warts, skin tags	Cuts / bruises / swellings/recent scars
Heart / Lung disorders	Varicose veins	Undiagnosed lumps /bumps
Cancer	Sunburn/Windburn	Recent hemorrhage
Pregnancy	Allergies, Asthma	Metal pins/plates
Thrombosis / Embolism	Skin disorders / diseases /active shingles	Swollen, hot or painful joints
Fractures / Sprains	Nerve dysfunction (e.g. MS)	Blood pressure disorders

ANY OTHER ISSUES THAT CONCERN YOU

OBJECTIVES OF THE TREATMENT & TREATMENT PLAN

What does the client hope to achieve?	
What will be possible to achieve realistically?	
Treatment plan agreed with the client (number of treatments to be given, over what period of time, length of time between treatments).	

PHYSICAL CONDITION OF THE CLIENT

Observations of the body during treatment (body type; condition of the skin, undiagnosed lumps/bumps, moles, varicose veins, scars, etc.)	
Initial findings after the session (did the client fully relax, was he/she talkative, nervous, any unusual observations, changes?)	

DISCLAIMER

I declare, that all the information regarding me in this form is true and accurate, and as far as I am aware, I can undertake a massage treatment without any adverse effects. I have been fully informed of any contra-indications and I am willing to undertake the treatment with this therapist.

Client's signature...Date...

AFTERCARE ADVICE

CLIENT FEEDBACK/ COMMENTS

Signature .... Date..

REFLEX POINTS – OBSERVATION NOTES
Image credit: https://vecteezy.com

REFLEXOLOGY CONSULTATION FORM

Therapist/ Clinic	Address, tel. number	Date

Client's Name	Gender	Doctor's name
Client's address	Age	Doctor's address
Tel. number	Occupation	Doctor's tel. number

GENERAL HEALTH

Symptoms presented by the client for treatment (if any)	General Health

LIFESTYLE/ BACKGROUND INFORMATION

Occupation	Stress level (1-10):	Diet:	Eating patterns
Family circumstances	Exercise	Fluid intake	Sleeping patterns
Relaxation	Alcohol intake	Smoker/non-smoker	Bowels

MEDICAL HISTORY

PAST MEDICAL HISTORY	PRESENT HEALTH
Recent operations	Medical conditions
Serious illnesses, accidents, injuries	Medication taken
Past treatments (received from other therapists or medical ones). When and why?	Current treatments

CONTRA-INDICATIONS/ CAUTIONS

Diabetes/Epilepsy	Arthritis / Rheumatism	Back / Neck Problems
Contagious/Infectious diseases	Moles (large, irregular), warts, skin tags	Cuts / bruises / swellings/recent scars
Heart / Lung disorders	Varicose veins	Undiagnosed lumps /bumps
Cancer	Sunburn/Windburn	Recent hemorrhage
Pregnancy	Allergies, Asthma	Metal pins/plates
Thrombosis / Embolism	Skin disorders / diseases /active shingles	Swollen, hot or painful joints
Fractures / Sprains	Nerve dysfunction (e.g. MS)	Blood pressure disorders

ANY OTHER ISSUES THAT CONCERN YOU

OBJECTIVES OF THE TREATMENT & TREATMENT PLAN

What does the client hope to achieve?	
What will be possible to achieve realistically?	
Treatment plan agreed with the client (number of treatments to be given, over what period of time, length of time between treatments).	

PHYSICAL CONDITION OF THE CLIENT

Observations of the body during treatment (body type; condition of the skin, undiagnosed lumps/bumps, moles, varicose veins, scars, etc.)	
Initial findings after the session (did the client fully relax, was he/she talkative, nervous, any unusual observations, changes?)	

DISCLAIMER

I declare, that all the information regarding me in this form is true and accurate, and as far as I am aware, I can undertake a massage treatment without any adverse effects. I have been fully informed of any contra-indications and I am willing to undertake the treatment with this therapist.

Client's signature..Date...

AFTERCARE ADVICE

CLIENT FEEDBACK/ COMMENTS

Signature .... Date...

REFLEX POINTS – OBSERVATION NOTES
Image credit: https://vecteezy.com

REFLEXOLOGY CONSULTATION FORM

Therapist/ Clinic	Address, tel. number	Date
Client's Name	Gender	Doctor's name
Client's address	Age	Doctor's address
Tel. number	Occupation	Doctor's tel. number

GENERAL HEALTH

Symptoms presented by the client for treatment (if any)	General Health

LIFESTYLE/ BACKGROUND INFORMATION

Occupation	Stress level (1-10):	Diet:	Eating patterns
Family circumstances	Exercise	Fluid intake	Sleeping patterns
Relaxation	Alcohol intake	Smoker/non-smoker	Bowels

MEDICAL HISTORY

PAST MEDICAL HISTORY	PRESENT HEALTH
Recent operations	Medical conditions
Serious illnesses, accidents, injuries	Medication taken
Past treatments (received from other therapists or medical ones). When and why?	Current treatments

CONTRA-INDICATIONS/ CAUTIONS

Diabetes/Epilepsy	Arthritis / Rheumatism	Back / Neck Problems
Contagious/Infectious diseases	Moles (large, irregular), warts, skin tags	Cuts / bruises / swellings/recent scars
Heart / Lung disorders	Varicose veins	Undiagnosed lumps /bumps
Cancer	Sunburn/Windburn	Recent hemorrhage
Pregnancy	Allergies, Asthma	Metal pins/plates
Thrombosis / Embolism	Skin disorders / diseases /active shingles	Swollen, hot or painful joints
Fractures / Sprains	Nerve dysfunction (e.g. MS)	Blood pressure disorders

ANY OTHER ISSUES THAT CONCERN YOU

OBJECTIVES OF THE TREATMENT & TREATMENT PLAN

What does the client hope to achieve?	
What will be possible to achieve realistically?	
Treatment plan agreed with the client (number of treatments to be given, over what period of time, length of time between treatments).	

PHYSICAL CONDITION OF THE CLIENT

Observations of the body during treatment (body type; condition of the skin, undiagnosed lumps/bumps, moles, varicose veins, scars, etc.)	
Initial findings after the session (did the client fully relax, was he/she talkative, nervous, any unusual observations, changes?)	

DISCLAIMER

I declare, that all the information regarding me in this form is true and accurate, and as far as I am aware, I can undertake a massage treatment without any adverse effects. I have been fully informed of any contra-indications and I am willing to undertake the treatment with this therapist.

Client's signature..Date..

AFTERCARE ADVICE

CLIENT FEEDBACK/ COMMENTS

Signature .... Date...

REFLEX POINTS – OBSERVATION NOTES
Image credit: https://vecteezy.com

REFLEXOLOGY CONSULTATION FORM

Therapist/ Clinic	Address, tel. number	Date
Client's Name	Gender	Doctor's name
Client's address	Age	Doctor's address
Tel. number	Occupation	Doctor's tel. number

GENERAL HEALTH

Symptoms presented by the client for treatment (if any)	General Health

LIFESTYLE/ BACKGROUND INFORMATION

Occupation	Stress level (1-10):	Diet:	Eating patterns
Family circumstances	Exercise	Fluid intake	Sleeping patterns
Relaxation	Alcohol intake	Smoker/non-smoker	Bowels

MEDICAL HISTORY

PAST MEDICAL HISTORY	PRESENT HEALTH
Recent operations	Medical conditions
Serious illnesses, accidents, injuries	Medication taken
Past treatments (received from other therapists or medical ones). When and why?	Current treatments

CONTRA-INDICATIONS/ CAUTIONS

Diabetes/Epilepsy	Arthritis / Rheumatism	Back / Neck Problems
Contagious/Infectious diseases	Moles (large, irregular), warts, skin tags	Cuts / bruises / swellings/recent scars
Heart / Lung disorders	Varicose veins	Undiagnosed lumps /bumps
Cancer	Sunburn/Windburn	Recent hemorrhage
Pregnancy	Allergies, Asthma	Metal pins/plates
Thrombosis / Embolism	Skin disorders / diseases /active shingles	Swollen, hot or painful joints
Fractures / Sprains	Nerve dysfunction (e.g. MS)	Blood pressure disorders

ANY OTHER ISSUES THAT CONCERN YOU

OBJECTIVES OF THE TREATMENT & TREATMENT PLAN

What does the client hope to achieve?	
What will be possible to achieve realistically?	
Treatment plan agreed with the client (number of treatments to be given, over what period of time, length of time between treatments).	

PHYSICAL CONDITION OF THE CLIENT

Observations of the body during treatment (body type; condition of the skin, undiagnosed lumps/bumps, moles, varicose veins, scars, etc.)	
Initial findings after the session (did the client fully relax, was he/she talkative, nervous, any unusual observations, changes?)	

DISCLAIMER

I declare, that all the information regarding me in this form is true and accurate, and as far as I am aware, I can undertake a massage treatment without any adverse effects. I have been fully informed of any contra-indications and I am willing to undertake the treatment with this therapist.

Client's signature...Date...

AFTERCARE ADVICE

CLIENT FEEDBACK/ COMMENTS

Signature .... Date..

REFLEX POINTS – OBSERVATION NOTES
Image credit: https://vecteezy.com

REFLEXOLOGY CONSULTATION FORM

Therapist/ Clinic	Address, tel. number	Date
Client's Name	Gender	Doctor's name
Client's address	Age	Doctor's address
Tel. number	Occupation	Doctor's tel. number

GENERAL HEALTH

Symptoms presented by the client for treatment (if any)	General Health

LIFESTYLE/ BACKGROUND INFORMATION

Occupation	Stress level (1-10):	Diet:	Eating patterns
Family circumstances	Exercise	Fluid intake	Sleeping patterns
Relaxation	Alcohol intake	Smoker/non-smoker	Bowels

MEDICAL HISTORY

PAST MEDICAL HISTORY	PRESENT HEALTH
Recent operations	Medical conditions
Serious illnesses, accidents, injuries	Medication taken
Past treatments (received from other therapists or medical ones). When and why?	Current treatments

CONTRA-INDICATIONS/ CAUTIONS

Diabetes/Epilepsy	Arthritis / Rheumatism	Back / Neck Problems
Contagious/Infectious diseases	Moles (large, irregular), warts, skin tags	Cuts / bruises / swellings/recent scars
Heart / Lung disorders	Varicose veins	Undiagnosed lumps /bumps
Cancer	Sunburn/Windburn	Recent hemorrhage
Pregnancy	Allergies, Asthma	Metal pins/plates
Thrombosis / Embolism	Skin disorders / diseases /active shingles	Swollen, hot or painful joints
Fractures / Sprains	Nerve dysfunction (e.g. MS)	Blood pressure disorders

ANY OTHER ISSUES THAT CONCERN YOU

OBJECTIVES OF THE TREATMENT & TREATMENT PLAN

What does the client hope to achieve?	
What will be possible to achieve realistically?	
Treatment plan agreed with the client (number of treatments to be given, over what period of time, length of time between treatments).	

PHYSICAL CONDITION OF THE CLIENT

Observations of the body during treatment (body type; condition of the skin, undiagnosed lumps/bumps, moles, varicose veins, scars, etc.)	
Initial findings after the session (did the client fully relax, was he/she talkative, nervous, any unusual observations, changes?)	

DISCLAIMER

I declare, that all the information regarding me in this form is true and accurate, and as far as I am aware, I can undertake a massage treatment without any adverse effects. I have been fully informed of any contra-indications and I am willing to undertake the treatment with this therapist.

Client's signature..Date..

AFTERCARE ADVICE

CLIENT FEEDBACK/ COMMENTS

Signature .... Date..

REFLEX POINTS – OBSERVATION NOTES
Image credit: https://vecteezy.com

REFLEXOLOGY CONSULTATION FORM

Therapist/ Clinic	Address, tel. number	Date
Client's Name	Gender	Doctor's name
Client's address	Age	Doctor's address
Tel. number	Occupation	Doctor's tel. number

GENERAL HEALTH

Symptoms presented by the client for treatment (if any)	General Health

LIFESTYLE/ BACKGROUND INFORMATION

Occupation	Stress level (1-10):	Diet:	Eating patterns
Family circumstances	Exercise	Fluid intake	Sleeping patterns
Relaxation	Alcohol intake	Smoker/non-smoker	Bowels

MEDICAL HISTORY

PAST MEDICAL HISTORY	PRESENT HEALTH
Recent operations	Medical conditions
Serious illnesses, accidents, injuries	Medication taken
Past treatments (received from other therapists or medical ones). When and why?	Current treatments

CONTRA-INDICATIONS/ CAUTIONS

Diabetes/Epilepsy	Arthritis / Rheumatism	Back / Neck Problems
Contagious/Infectious diseases	Moles (large, irregular), warts, skin tags	Cuts / bruises / swellings/recent scars
Heart / Lung disorders	Varicose veins	Undiagnosed lumps /bumps
Cancer	Sunburn/Windburn	Recent hemorrhage
Pregnancy	Allergies, Asthma	Metal pins/plates
Thrombosis / Embolism	Skin disorders / diseases /active shingles	Swollen, hot or painful joints
Fractures / Sprains	Nerve dysfunction (e.g. MS)	Blood pressure disorders

ANY OTHER ISSUES THAT CONCERN YOU

OBJECTIVES OF THE TREATMENT & TREATMENT PLAN

What does the client hope to achieve?	
What will be possible to achieve realistically?	
Treatment plan agreed with the client (number of treatments to be given, over what period of time, length of time between treatments).	

PHYSICAL CONDITION OF THE CLIENT

Observations of the body during treatment (body type; condition of the skin, undiagnosed lumps/bumps, moles, varicose veins, scars, etc.)	
Initial findings after the session (did the client fully relax, was he/she talkative, nervous, any unusual observations, changes?)	

DISCLAIMER

I declare, that all the information regarding me in this form is true and accurate, and as far as I am aware, I can undertake a massage treatment without any adverse effects. I have been fully informed of any contra-indications and I am willing to undertake the treatment with this therapist.

Client's signature...Date..

AFTERCARE ADVICE

CLIENT FEEDBACK/ COMMENTS

Signature .... Date..

REFLEX POINTS – OBSERVATION NOTES

Image credit: https://vecteezy.com

REFLEXOLOGY CONSULTATION FORM

Therapist/ Clinic	Address, tel. number	Date
Client's Name	Gender	Doctor's name
Client's address	Age	Doctor's address
Tel. number	Occupation	Doctor's tel. number

GENERAL HEALTH

Symptoms presented by the client for treatment (if any)	General Health

LIFESTYLE/ BACKGROUND INFORMATION

Occupation	Stress level (1-10):	Diet:	Eating patterns
Family circumstances	Exercise	Fluid intake	Sleeping patterns
Relaxation	Alcohol intake	Smoker/non-smoker	Bowels

MEDICAL HISTORY

PAST MEDICAL HISTORY	PRESENT HEALTH
Recent operations	Medical conditions
Serious illnesses, accidents, injuries	Medication taken
Past treatments (received from other therapists or medical ones). When and why?	Current treatments

CONTRA-INDICATIONS/ CAUTIONS

Diabetes/Epilepsy	Arthritis / Rheumatism	Back / Neck Problems
Contagious/Infectious diseases	Moles (large, irregular), warts, skin tags	Cuts / bruises / swellings/recent scars
Heart / Lung disorders	Varicose veins	Undiagnosed lumps /bumps
Cancer	Sunburn/Windburn	Recent hemorrhage
Pregnancy	Allergies, Asthma	Metal pins/plates
Thrombosis / Embolism	Skin disorders / diseases /active shingles	Swollen, hot or painful joints
Fractures / Sprains	Nerve dysfunction (e.g. MS)	Blood pressure disorders

ANY OTHER ISSUES THAT CONCERN YOU

OBJECTIVES OF THE TREATMENT & TREATMENT PLAN

What does the client hope to achieve?	
What will be possible to achieve realistically?	
Treatment plan agreed with the client (number of treatments to be given, over what period of time, length of time between treatments).	

PHYSICAL CONDITION OF THE CLIENT

Observations of the body during treatment (body type; condition of the skin, undiagnosed lumps/bumps, moles, varicose veins, scars, etc.)	
Initial findings after the session (did the client fully relax, was he/she talkative, nervous, any unusual observations, changes?)	

DISCLAIMER

I declare, that all the information regarding me in this form is true and accurate, and as far as I am aware, I can undertake a massage treatment without any adverse effects. I have been fully informed of any contra-indications and I am willing to undertake the treatment with this therapist.

Client's signature...Date...

AFTERCARE ADVICE

CLIENT FEEDBACK/ COMMENTS

Signature .... Date...

REFLEX POINTS – OBSERVATION NOTES
Image credit: https://vecteezy.com

REFLEXOLOGY CONSULTATION FORM

Therapist/ Clinic	Address, tel. number	Date
Client's Name	Gender	Doctor's name
Client's address	Age	Doctor's address
Tel. number	Occupation	Doctor's tel. number

GENERAL HEALTH

Symptoms presented by the client for treatment (if any)	General Health

LIFESTYLE/ BACKGROUND INFORMATION

Occupation	Stress level (1-10):	Diet:	Eating patterns
Family circumstances	Exercise	Fluid intake	Sleeping patterns
Relaxation	Alcohol intake	Smoker/non-smoker	Bowels

MEDICAL HISTORY

PAST MEDICAL HISTORY	PRESENT HEALTH
Recent operations	Medical conditions
Serious illnesses, accidents, injuries	Medication taken
Past treatments (received from other therapists or medical ones). When and why?	Current treatments

CONTRA-INDICATIONS/ CAUTIONS

Diabetes/Epilepsy	Arthritis / Rheumatism	Back / Neck Problems
Contagious/Infectious diseases	Moles (large, irregular), warts, skin tags	Cuts / bruises / swellings/recent scars
Heart / Lung disorders	Varicose veins	Undiagnosed lumps /bumps
Cancer	Sunburn/Windburn	Recent hemorrhage
Pregnancy	Allergies, Asthma	Metal pins/plates
Thrombosis / Embolism	Skin disorders / diseases /active shingles	Swollen, hot or painful joints
Fractures / Sprains	Nerve dysfunction (e.g. MS)	Blood pressure disorders

ANY OTHER ISSUES THAT CONCERN YOU

OBJECTIVES OF THE TREATMENT & TREATMENT PLAN

What does the client hope to achieve?	
What will be possible to achieve realistically?	
Treatment plan agreed with the client (number of treatments to be given, over what period of time, length of time between treatments).	

PHYSICAL CONDITION OF THE CLIENT

Observations of the body during treatment (body type; condition of the skin, undiagnosed lumps/bumps, moles, varicose veins, scars, etc.)	
Initial findings after the session (did the client fully relax, was he/she talkative, nervous, any unusual observations, changes?)	

DISCLAIMER

I declare, that all the information regarding me in this form is true and accurate, and as far as I am aware, I can undertake a massage treatment without any adverse effects. I have been fully informed of any contra-indications and I am willing to undertake the treatment with this therapist.

Client's signature...Date...

AFTERCARE ADVICE

CLIENT FEEDBACK/ COMMENTS

Signature .... Date...

REFLEX POINTS – OBSERVATION NOTES

Image credit: https://vecteezy.com

REFLEXOLOGY CONSULTATION FORM

Therapist/ Clinic	Address, tel. number	Date
Client's Name	Gender	Doctor's name
Client's address	Age	Doctor's address
Tel. number	Occupation	Doctor's tel. number

GENERAL HEALTH

Symptoms presented by the client for treatment (if any)	General Health

LIFESTYLE/ BACKGROUND INFORMATION

Occupation	Stress level (1-10):	Diet:	Eating patterns
Family circumstances	Exercise	Fluid intake	Sleeping patterns
Relaxation	Alcohol intake	Smoker/non-smoker	Bowels

MEDICAL HISTORY

PAST MEDICAL HISTORY	PRESENT HEALTH
Recent operations	Medical conditions
Serious illnesses, accidents, injuries	Medication taken
Past treatments (received from other therapists or medical ones). When and why?	Current treatments

CONTRA-INDICATIONS/ CAUTIONS

Diabetes/Epilepsy	Arthritis / Rheumatism	Back / Neck Problems
Contagious/Infectious diseases	Moles (large, irregular), warts, skin tags	Cuts / bruises / swellings/recent scars
Heart / Lung disorders	Varicose veins	Undiagnosed lumps /bumps
Cancer	Sunburn/Windburn	Recent hemorrhage
Pregnancy	Allergies, Asthma	Metal pins/plates
Thrombosis / Embolism	Skin disorders / diseases /active shingles	Swollen, hot or painful joints
Fractures / Sprains	Nerve dysfunction (e.g. MS)	Blood pressure disorders

ANY OTHER ISSUES THAT CONCERN YOU

OBJECTIVES OF THE TREATMENT & TREATMENT PLAN

What does the client hope to achieve?	
What will be possible to achieve realistically?	
Treatment plan agreed with the client (number of treatments to be given, over what period of time, length of time between treatments).	

PHYSICAL CONDITION OF THE CLIENT

Observations of the body during treatment (body type; condition of the skin, undiagnosed lumps/bumps, moles, varicose veins, scars, etc.)	
Initial findings after the session (did the client fully relax, was he/she talkative, nervous, any unusual observations, changes?)	

DISCLAIMER

I declare, that all the information regarding me in this form is true and accurate, and as far as I am aware, I can undertake a massage treatment without any adverse effects. I have been fully informed of any contra-indications and I am willing to undertake the treatment with this therapist.

Client's signature...Date..

AFTERCARE ADVICE

CLIENT FEEDBACK/ COMMENTS

Signature .... Date...

REFLEX POINTS – OBSERVATION NOTES
Image credit: https://vecteezy.com

REFLEXOLOGY CONSULTATION FORM

Therapist/ Clinic	Address, tel. number	Date
Client's Name	Gender	Doctor's name
Client's address	Age	Doctor's address
Tel. number	Occupation	Doctor's tel. number

GENERAL HEALTH

Symptoms presented by the client for treatment (if any)	General Health

LIFESTYLE/ BACKGROUND INFORMATION

Occupation	Stress level (1-10):	Diet:	Eating patterns
Family circumstances	Exercise	Fluid intake	Sleeping patterns
Relaxation	Alcohol intake	Smoker/non-smoker	Bowels

MEDICAL HISTORY

PAST MEDICAL HISTORY	PRESENT HEALTH
Recent operations	Medical conditions
Serious illnesses, accidents, injuries	Medication taken
Past treatments (received from other therapists or medical ones). When and why?	Current treatments

CONTRA-INDICATIONS/ CAUTIONS

Diabetes/Epilepsy	Arthritis / Rheumatism	Back / Neck Problems
Contagious/Infectious diseases	Moles (large, irregular), warts, skin tags	Cuts / bruises / swellings/recent scars
Heart / Lung disorders	Varicose veins	Undiagnosed lumps /bumps
Cancer	Sunburn/Windburn	Recent hemorrhage
Pregnancy	Allergies, Asthma	Metal pins/plates
Thrombosis / Embolism	Skin disorders / diseases /active shingles	Swollen, hot or painful joints
Fractures / Sprains	Nerve dysfunction (e.g. MS)	Blood pressure disorders

ANY OTHER ISSUES THAT CONCERN YOU

OBJECTIVES OF THE TREATMENT & TREATMENT PLAN

What does the client hope to achieve?	
What will be possible to achieve realistically?	
Treatment plan agreed with the client (number of treatments to be given, over what period of time, length of time between treatments).	

PHYSICAL CONDITION OF THE CLIENT

Observations of the body during treatment (body type; condition of the skin, undiagnosed lumps/bumps, moles, varicose veins, scars, etc.)	
Initial findings after the session (did the client fully relax, was he/she talkative, nervous, any unusual observations, changes?)	

DISCLAIMER

I declare, that all the information regarding me in this form is true and accurate, and as far as I am aware, I can undertake a massage treatment without any adverse effects. I have been fully informed of any contra-indications and I am willing to undertake the treatment with this therapist.

Client's signature...Date...

AFTERCARE ADVICE

CLIENT FEEDBACK/ COMMENTS

Signature .... Date...

REFLEX POINTS – OBSERVATION NOTES

Image credit: https://vecteezy.com

REFLEXOLOGY CONSULTATION FORM

Therapist/ Clinic	Address, tel. number		Date
Client's Name	Gender	Doctor's name	
Client's address	Age	Doctor's address	
Tel. number	Occupation	Doctor's tel. number	

GENERAL HEALTH

Symptoms presented by the client for treatment (if any)	General Health

LIFESTYLE/ BACKGROUND INFORMATION

Occupation	Stress level (1-10):	Diet:	Eating patterns
Family circumstances	Exercise	Fluid intake	Sleeping patterns
Relaxation	Alcohol intake	Smoker/non-smoker	Bowels

MEDICAL HISTORY

PAST MEDICAL HISTORY	PRESENT HEALTH
Recent operations	Medical conditions
Serious illnesses, accidents, injuries	Medication taken
Past treatments (received from other therapists or medical ones). When and why?	Current treatments

CONTRA-INDICATIONS/ CAUTIONS

Diabetes/Epilepsy	Arthritis / Rheumatism	Back / Neck Problems
Contagious/Infectious diseases	Moles (large, irregular), warts, skin tags	Cuts / bruises / swellings/recent scars
Heart / Lung disorders	Varicose veins	Undiagnosed lumps /bumps
Cancer	Sunburn/Windburn	Recent hemorrhage
Pregnancy	Allergies, Asthma	Metal pins/plates
Thrombosis / Embolism	Skin disorders / diseases /active shingles	Swollen, hot or painful joints
Fractures / Sprains	Nerve dysfunction (e.g. MS)	Blood pressure disorders

ANY OTHER ISSUES THAT CONCERN YOU

OBJECTIVES OF THE TREATMENT & TREATMENT PLAN

What does the client hope to achieve?	
What will be possible to achieve realistically?	
Treatment plan agreed with the client (number of treatments to be given, over what period of time, length of time between treatments).	

PHYSICAL CONDITION OF THE CLIENT

Observations of the body during treatment (body type; condition of the skin, undiagnosed lumps/bumps, moles, varicose veins, scars, etc.)	
Initial findings after the session (did the client fully relax, was he/she talkative, nervous, any unusual observations, changes?)	

DISCLAIMER

I declare, that all the information regarding me in this form is true and accurate, and as far as I am aware, I can undertake a massage treatment without any adverse effects. I have been fully informed of any contra-indications and I am willing to undertake the treatment with this therapist.

Client's signature...Date...

AFTERCARE ADVICE

CLIENT FEEDBACK/ COMMENTS

Signature .... Date...

REFLEX POINTS – OBSERVATION NOTES
Image credit: https://vecteezy.com

REFLEXOLOGY CONSULTATION FORM

Therapist/ Clinic	Address, tel. number	Date
Client's Name Client's address Tel. number	Gender Age Occupation	Doctor's name Doctor's address Doctor's tel. number

GENERAL HEALTH

Symptoms presented by the client for treatment (if any)	General Health

LIFESTYLE/ BACKGROUND INFORMATION

Occupation	Stress level (1-10):	Diet:	Eating patterns
Family circumstances	Exercise	Fluid intake	Sleeping patterns
Relaxation	Alcohol intake	Smoker/non-smoker	Bowels

MEDICAL HISTORY

PAST MEDICAL HISTORY	PRESENT HEALTH
Recent operations	Medical conditions
Serious illnesses, accidents, injuries	Medication taken
Past treatments (received from other therapists or medical ones). When and why?	Current treatments

CONTRA-INDICATIONS/ CAUTIONS

Diabetes/Epilepsy	Arthritis / Rheumatism	Back / Neck Problems
Contagious/Infectious diseases	Moles (large, irregular), warts, skin tags	Cuts / bruises / swellings/recent scars
Heart / Lung disorders	Varicose veins	Undiagnosed lumps /bumps
Cancer	Sunburn/Windburn	Recent hemorrhage
Pregnancy	Allergies, Asthma	Metal pins/plates
Thrombosis / Embolism	Skin disorders / diseases /active shingles	Swollen, hot or painful joints
Fractures / Sprains	Nerve dysfunction (e.g. MS)	Blood pressure disorders

ANY OTHER ISSUES THAT CONCERN YOU

OBJECTIVES OF THE TREATMENT & TREATMENT PLAN

What does the client hope to achieve?	
What will be possible to achieve realistically?	
Treatment plan agreed with the client (number of treatments to be given, over what period of time, length of time between treatments).	

PHYSICAL CONDITION OF THE CLIENT

Observations of the body during treatment (body type; condition of the skin, undiagnosed lumps/bumps, moles, varicose veins, scars, etc.)	
Initial findings after the session (did the client fully relax, was he/she talkative, nervous, any unusual observations, changes?)	

DISCLAIMER

I declare, that all the information regarding me in this form is true and accurate, and as far as I am aware, I can undertake a massage treatment without any adverse effects. I have been fully informed of any contra-indications and I am willing to undertake the treatment with this therapist.

Client's signature...Date...

AFTERCARE ADVICE

CLIENT FEEDBACK/ COMMENTS

Signature .... Date...

REFLEX POINTS – OBSERVATION NOTES
Image credit: https://vecteezy.com

REFLEXOLOGY CONSULTATION FORM

Therapist/ Clinic	Address, tel. number	Date
Client's Name	Gender	Doctor's name
Client's address	Age	Doctor's address
Tel. number	Occupation	Doctor's tel. number

GENERAL HEALTH

Symptoms presented by the client for treatment (if any)	General Health

LIFESTYLE/ BACKGROUND INFORMATION

Occupation	Stress level (1-10):	Diet:	Eating patterns
Family circumstances	Exercise	Fluid intake	Sleeping patterns
Relaxation	Alcohol intake	Smoker/non-smoker	Bowels

MEDICAL HISTORY

PAST MEDICAL HISTORY	PRESENT HEALTH
Recent operations	Medical conditions
Serious illnesses, accidents, injuries	Medication taken
Past treatments (received from other therapists or medical ones). When and why?	Current treatments

CONTRA-INDICATIONS/ CAUTIONS

Diabetes/Epilepsy	Arthritis / Rheumatism	Back / Neck Problems
Contagious/Infectious diseases	Moles (large, irregular), warts, skin tags	Cuts / bruises / swellings/recent scars
Heart / Lung disorders	Varicose veins	Undiagnosed lumps /bumps
Cancer	Sunburn/Windburn	Recent hemorrhage
Pregnancy	Allergies, Asthma	Metal pins/plates
Thrombosis / Embolism	Skin disorders / diseases /active shingles	Swollen, hot or painful joints
Fractures / Sprains	Nerve dysfunction (e.g. MS)	Blood pressure disorders

ANY OTHER ISSUES THAT CONCERN YOU

OBJECTIVES OF THE TREATMENT & TREATMENT PLAN

What does the client hope to achieve?	
What will be possible to achieve realistically?	
Treatment plan agreed with the client (number of treatments to be given, over what period of time, length of time between treatments).	

PHYSICAL CONDITION OF THE CLIENT

Observations of the body during treatment (body type; condition of the skin, undiagnosed lumps/bumps, moles, varicose veins, scars, etc.)	
Initial findings after the session (did the client fully relax, was he/she talkative, nervous, any unusual observations, changes?)	

DISCLAIMER

I declare, that all the information regarding me in this form is true and accurate, and as far as I am aware, I can undertake a massage treatment without any adverse effects. I have been fully informed of any contra-indications and I am willing to undertake the treatment with this therapist.

Client's signature...Date..

AFTERCARE ADVICE

CLIENT FEEDBACK/ COMMENTS

Signature .... Date..

REFLEX POINTS – OBSERVATION NOTES
Image credit: https://vecteezy.com

REFLEXOLOGY CONSULTATION FORM

Therapist/ Clinic	Address, tel. number	Date
Client's Name	Gender	Doctor's name
Client's address	Age	Doctor's address
Tel. number	Occupation	Doctor's tel. number

GENERAL HEALTH

Symptoms presented by the client for treatment (if any)	General Health

LIFESTYLE/ BACKGROUND INFORMATION

Occupation	Stress level (1-10):	Diet:	Eating patterns
Family circumstances	Exercise	Fluid intake	Sleeping patterns
Relaxation	Alcohol intake	Smoker/non-smoker	Bowels

MEDICAL HISTORY

PAST MEDICAL HISTORY	PRESENT HEALTH
Recent operations	Medical conditions
Serious illnesses, accidents, injuries	Medication taken
Past treatments (received from other therapists or medical ones). When and why?	Current treatments

CONTRA-INDICATIONS/ CAUTIONS

Diabetes/Epilepsy	Arthritis / Rheumatism	Back / Neck Problems
Contagious/Infectious diseases	Moles (large, irregular), warts, skin tags	Cuts / bruises / swellings/recent scars
Heart / Lung disorders	Varicose veins	Undiagnosed lumps /bumps
Cancer	Sunburn/Windburn	Recent hemorrhage
Pregnancy	Allergies, Asthma	Metal pins/plates
Thrombosis / Embolism	Skin disorders / diseases /active shingles	Swollen, hot or painful joints
Fractures / Sprains	Nerve dysfunction (e.g. MS)	Blood pressure disorders

ANY OTHER ISSUES THAT CONCERN YOU

OBJECTIVES OF THE TREATMENT & TREATMENT PLAN

What does the client hope to achieve?	
What will be possible to achieve realistically?	
Treatment plan agreed with the client (number of treatments to be given, over what period of time, length of time between treatments).	

PHYSICAL CONDITION OF THE CLIENT

Observations of the body during treatment (body type; condition of the skin, undiagnosed lumps/bumps, moles, varicose veins, scars, etc.)	
Initial findings after the session (did the client fully relax, was he/she talkative, nervous, any unusual observations, changes?)	

DISCLAIMER

I declare, that all the information regarding me in this form is true and accurate, and as far as I am aware, I can undertake a massage treatment without any adverse effects. I have been fully informed of any contra-indications and I am willing to undertake the treatment with this therapist.

Client's signature...Date...

AFTERCARE ADVICE

CLIENT FEEDBACK/ COMMENTS

Signature .... Date...

REFLEX POINTS – OBSERVATION NOTES

Image credit: https://vecteezy.com

REFLEXOLOGY CONSULTATION FORM

Therapist/ Clinic	Address, tel. number	Date
Client's Name	Gender	Doctor's name
Client's address	Age	Doctor's address
Tel. number	Occupation	Doctor's tel. number

GENERAL HEALTH

Symptoms presented by the client for treatment (if any)	General Health

LIFESTYLE/ BACKGROUND INFORMATION

Occupation	Stress level (1-10):	Diet:	Eating patterns
Family circumstances	Exercise	Fluid intake	Sleeping patterns
Relaxation	Alcohol intake	Smoker/non-smoker	Bowels

MEDICAL HISTORY

PAST MEDICAL HISTORY	PRESENT HEALTH
Recent operations	Medical conditions
Serious illnesses, accidents, injuries	Medication taken
Past treatments (received from other therapists or medical ones). When and why?	Current treatments

CONTRA-INDICATIONS/ CAUTIONS

Diabetes/Epilepsy	Arthritis / Rheumatism	Back / Neck Problems
Contagious/Infectious diseases	Moles (large, irregular), warts, skin tags	Cuts / bruises / swellings/recent scars
Heart / Lung disorders	Varicose veins	Undiagnosed lumps /bumps
Cancer	Sunburn/Windburn	Recent hemorrhage
Pregnancy	Allergies, Asthma	Metal pins/plates
Thrombosis / Embolism	Skin disorders / diseases /active shingles	Swollen, hot or painful joints
Fractures / Sprains	Nerve dysfunction (e.g. MS)	Blood pressure disorders

ANY OTHER ISSUES THAT CONCERN YOU

OBJECTIVES OF THE TREATMENT & TREATMENT PLAN

What does the client hope to achieve?	
What will be possible to achieve realistically?	
Treatment plan agreed with the client (number of treatments to be given, over what period of time, length of time between treatments).	

PHYSICAL CONDITION OF THE CLIENT

Observations of the body during treatment (body type; condition of the skin, undiagnosed lumps/bumps, moles, varicose veins, scars, etc.)	
Initial findings after the session (did the client fully relax, was he/she talkative, nervous, any unusual observations, changes?)	

DISCLAIMER

I declare, that all the information regarding me in this form is true and accurate, and as far as I am aware, I can undertake a massage treatment without any adverse effects. I have been fully informed of any contra-indications and I am willing to undertake the treatment with this therapist.

Client's signature...Date..

AFTERCARE ADVICE

CLIENT FEEDBACK/ COMMENTS

Signature .... Date..

REFLEX POINTS – OBSERVATION NOTES
Image credit: https://vecteezy.com

REFLEXOLOGY CONSULTATION FORM

Therapist/ Clinic	Address, tel. number	Date
Client's Name	Gender	Doctor's name
Client's address	Age	Doctor's address
Tel. number	Occupation	Doctor's tel. number

GENERAL HEALTH

Symptoms presented by the client for treatment (if any)	General Health

LIFESTYLE/ BACKGROUND INFORMATION

Occupation	Stress level (1-10):	Diet:	Eating patterns
Family circumstances	Exercise	Fluid intake	Sleeping patterns
Relaxation	Alcohol intake	Smoker/non-smoker	Bowels

MEDICAL HISTORY

PAST MEDICAL HISTORY	PRESENT HEALTH
Recent operations	Medical conditions
Serious illnesses, accidents, injuries	Medication taken
Past treatments (received from other therapists or medical ones). When and why?	Current treatments

CONTRA-INDICATIONS/ CAUTIONS

Diabetes/Epilepsy	Arthritis / Rheumatism	Back / Neck Problems
Contagious/Infectious diseases	Moles (large, irregular), warts, skin tags	Cuts / bruises / swellings/recent scars
Heart / Lung disorders	Varicose veins	Undiagnosed lumps /bumps
Cancer	Sunburn/Windburn	Recent hemorrhage
Pregnancy	Allergies, Asthma	Metal pins/plates
Thrombosis / Embolism	Skin disorders / diseases /active shingles	Swollen, hot or painful joints
Fractures / Sprains	Nerve dysfunction (e.g. MS)	Blood pressure disorders

ANY OTHER ISSUES THAT CONCERN YOU

OBJECTIVES OF THE TREATMENT & TREATMENT PLAN

What does the client hope to achieve?	
What will be possible to achieve realistically?	
Treatment plan agreed with the client (number of treatments to be given, over what period of time, length of time between treatments).	

PHYSICAL CONDITION OF THE CLIENT

Observations of the body during treatment (body type; condition of the skin, undiagnosed lumps/bumps, moles, varicose veins, scars, etc.)	
Initial findings after the session (did the client fully relax, was he/she talkative, nervous, any unusual observations, changes?)	

DISCLAIMER

I declare, that all the information regarding me in this form is true and accurate, and as far as I am aware, I can undertake a massage treatment without any adverse effects. I have been fully informed of any contra-indications and I am willing to undertake the treatment with this therapist.

Client's signature..Date...

AFTERCARE ADVICE

CLIENT FEEDBACK/ COMMENTS

Signature .... Date...

REFLEX POINTS – OBSERVATION NOTES
Image credit: https://vecteezy.com

REFLEXOLOGY CONSULTATION FORM

Therapist/ Clinic	Address, tel. number	Date
Client's Name	Gender	Doctor's name
Client's address	Age	Doctor's address
Tel. number	Occupation	Doctor's tel. number

GENERAL HEALTH

Symptoms presented by the client for treatment (if any)	General Health

LIFESTYLE/ BACKGROUND INFORMATION

Occupation	Stress level (1-10):	Diet:	Eating patterns
Family circumstances	Exercise	Fluid intake	Sleeping patterns
Relaxation	Alcohol intake	Smoker/non-smoker	Bowels

MEDICAL HISTORY

PAST MEDICAL HISTORY	PRESENT HEALTH
Recent operations	Medical conditions
Serious illnesses, accidents, injuries	Medication taken
Past treatments (received from other therapists or medical ones). When and why?	Current treatments

CONTRA-INDICATIONS/ CAUTIONS

Diabetes/Epilepsy	Arthritis / Rheumatism	Back / Neck Problems
Contagious/Infectious diseases	Moles (large, irregular), warts, skin tags	Cuts / bruises / swellings/recent scars
Heart / Lung disorders	Varicose veins	Undiagnosed lumps /bumps
Cancer	Sunburn/Windburn	Recent hemorrhage
Pregnancy	Allergies, Asthma	Metal pins/plates
Thrombosis / Embolism	Skin disorders / diseases /active shingles	Swollen, hot or painful joints
Fractures / Sprains	Nerve dysfunction (e.g. MS)	Blood pressure disorders

ANY OTHER ISSUES THAT CONCERN YOU

OBJECTIVES OF THE TREATMENT & TREATMENT PLAN

What does the client hope to achieve?	
What will be possible to achieve realistically?	
Treatment plan agreed with the client (number of treatments to be given, over what period of time, length of time between treatments).	

PHYSICAL CONDITION OF THE CLIENT

Observations of the body during treatment (body type; condition of the skin, undiagnosed lumps/bumps, moles, varicose veins, scars, etc.)	
Initial findings after the session (did the client fully relax, was he/she talkative, nervous, any unusual observations, changes?)	

DISCLAIMER

I declare, that all the information regarding me in this form is true and accurate, and as far as I am aware, I can undertake a massage treatment without any adverse effects. I have been fully informed of any contra-indications and I am willing to undertake the treatment with this therapist.

Client's signature...Date...

AFTERCARE ADVICE

CLIENT FEEDBACK/ COMMENTS

Signature .... Date...

REFLEX POINTS – OBSERVATION NOTES
Image credit: https://vecteezy.com

REFLEXOLOGY CONSULTATION FORM

Therapist/ Clinic	Address, tel. number	Date
Client's Name	Gender	Doctor's name
Client's address	Age	Doctor's address
Tel. number	Occupation	Doctor's tel. number

GENERAL HEALTH

Symptoms presented by the client for treatment (if any)	General Health

LIFESTYLE/ BACKGROUND INFORMATION

Occupation	Stress level (1-10):	Diet:	Eating patterns
Family circumstances	Exercise	Fluid intake	Sleeping patterns
Relaxation	Alcohol intake	Smoker/non-smoker	Bowels

MEDICAL HISTORY

PAST MEDICAL HISTORY	PRESENT HEALTH
Recent operations	Medical conditions
Serious illnesses, accidents, injuries	Medication taken
Past treatments (received from other therapists or medical ones). When and why?	Current treatments

CONTRA-INDICATIONS/ CAUTIONS

Diabetes/Epilepsy	Arthritis / Rheumatism	Back / Neck Problems
Contagious/Infectious diseases	Moles (large, irregular), warts, skin tags	Cuts / bruises / swellings/recent scars
Heart / Lung disorders	Varicose veins	Undiagnosed lumps /bumps
Cancer	Sunburn/Windburn	Recent hemorrhage
Pregnancy	Allergies, Asthma	Metal pins/plates
Thrombosis / Embolism	Skin disorders / diseases /active shingles	Swollen, hot or painful joints
Fractures / Sprains	Nerve dysfunction (e.g. MS)	Blood pressure disorders

ANY OTHER ISSUES THAT CONCERN YOU

OBJECTIVES OF THE TREATMENT & TREATMENT PLAN

What does the client hope to achieve?	
What will be possible to achieve realistically?	
Treatment plan agreed with the client (number of treatments to be given, over what period of time, length of time between treatments).	

PHYSICAL CONDITION OF THE CLIENT

Observations of the body during treatment (body type; condition of the skin, undiagnosed lumps/bumps, moles, varicose veins, scars, etc.)	
Initial findings after the session (did the client fully relax, was he/she talkative, nervous, any unusual observations, changes?)	

DISCLAIMER

I declare, that all the information regarding me in this form is true and accurate, and as far as I am aware, I can undertake a massage treatment without any adverse effects. I have been fully informed of any contra-indications and I am willing to undertake the treatment with this therapist.

Client's signature...Date...

AFTERCARE ADVICE

CLIENT FEEDBACK/ COMMENTS

Signature .... Date...

REFLEX POINTS – OBSERVATION NOTES
Image credit: https://vecteezy.com

REFLEXOLOGY CONSULTATION FORM

Therapist/ Clinic	Address, tel. number	Date
Client's Name Client's address Tel. number	Gender Age Occupation	Doctor's name Doctor's address Doctor's tel. number

GENERAL HEALTH

Symptoms presented by the client for treatment (if any)	General Health

LIFESTYLE/ BACKGROUND INFORMATION

Occupation	Stress level (1-10):	Diet:	Eating patterns
Family circumstances	Exercise	Fluid intake	Sleeping patterns
Relaxation	Alcohol intake	Smoker/non-smoker	Bowels

MEDICAL HISTORY

PAST MEDICAL HISTORY	PRESENT HEALTH
Recent operations	Medical conditions
Serious illnesses, accidents, injuries	Medication taken
Past treatments (received from other therapists or medical ones). When and why?	Current treatments

CONTRA-INDICATIONS/ CAUTIONS

Diabetes/Epilepsy	Arthritis / Rheumatism	Back / Neck Problems
Contagious/Infectious diseases	Moles (large, irregular), warts, skin tags	Cuts / bruises / swellings/recent scars
Heart / Lung disorders	Varicose veins	Undiagnosed lumps /bumps
Cancer	Sunburn/Windburn	Recent hemorrhage
Pregnancy	Allergies, Asthma	Metal pins/plates
Thrombosis / Embolism	Skin disorders / diseases /active shingles	Swollen, hot or painful joints
Fractures / Sprains	Nerve dysfunction (e.g. MS)	Blood pressure disorders

ANY OTHER ISSUES THAT CONCERN YOU

OBJECTIVES OF THE TREATMENT & TREATMENT PLAN

What does the client hope to achieve?	
What will be possible to achieve realistically?	
Treatment plan agreed with the client (number of treatments to be given, over what period of time, length of time between treatments).	

PHYSICAL CONDITION OF THE CLIENT

Observations of the body during treatment (body type; condition of the skin, undiagnosed lumps/bumps, moles, varicose veins, scars, etc.)	
Initial findings after the session (did the client fully relax, was he/she talkative, nervous, any unusual observations, changes?)	

DISCLAIMER

I declare, that all the information regarding me in this form is true and accurate, and as far as I am aware, I can undertake a massage treatment without any adverse effects. I have been fully informed of any contra-indications and I am willing to undertake the treatment with this therapist.

Client's signature...Date...

AFTERCARE ADVICE

CLIENT FEEDBACK/ COMMENTS

Signature .... Date..

REFLEX POINTS – OBSERVATION NOTES
Image credit: https://vecteezy.com

REFLEXOLOGY CONSULTATION FORM

Therapist/ Clinic	Address, tel. number	Date
Client's Name	Gender	Doctor's name
Client's address	Age	Doctor's address
Tel. number	Occupation	Doctor's tel. number

GENERAL HEALTH

Symptoms presented by the client for treatment (if any)	General Health

LIFESTYLE/ BACKGROUND INFORMATION

Occupation	Stress level (1-10):	Diet:	Eating patterns
Family circumstances	Exercise	Fluid intake	Sleeping patterns
Relaxation	Alcohol intake	Smoker/non-smoker	Bowels

MEDICAL HISTORY

PAST MEDICAL HISTORY	PRESENT HEALTH
Recent operations	Medical conditions
Serious illnesses, accidents, injuries	Medication taken
Past treatments (received from other therapists or medical ones). When and why?	Current treatments

CONTRA-INDICATIONS/ CAUTIONS

Diabetes/Epilepsy	Arthritis / Rheumatism	Back / Neck Problems
Contagious/Infectious diseases	Moles (large, irregular), warts, skin tags	Cuts / bruises / swellings/recent scars
Heart / Lung disorders	Varicose veins	Undiagnosed lumps /bumps
Cancer	Sunburn/Windburn	Recent hemorrhage
Pregnancy	Allergies, Asthma	Metal pins/plates
Thrombosis / Embolism	Skin disorders / diseases /active shingles	Swollen, hot or painful joints
Fractures / Sprains	Nerve dysfunction (e.g. MS)	Blood pressure disorders

ANY OTHER ISSUES THAT CONCERN YOU

OBJECTIVES OF THE TREATMENT & TREATMENT PLAN

What does the client hope to achieve?	
What will be possible to achieve realistically?	
Treatment plan agreed with the client (number of treatments to be given, over what period of time, length of time between treatments).	

PHYSICAL CONDITION OF THE CLIENT

Observations of the body during treatment (body type; condition of the skin, undiagnosed lumps/bumps, moles, varicose veins, scars, etc.)	
Initial findings after the session (did the client fully relax, was he/she talkative, nervous, any unusual observations, changes?)	

DISCLAIMER

I declare, that all the information regarding me in this form is true and accurate, and as far as I am aware, I can undertake a massage treatment without any adverse effects. I have been fully informed of any contra-indications and I am willing to undertake the treatment with this therapist.

Client's signature...Date...

AFTERCARE ADVICE

CLIENT FEEDBACK/ COMMENTS

Signature .... Date..

REFLEX POINTS – OBSERVATION NOTES
Image credit: https://vecteezy.com

REFLEXOLOGY CONSULTATION FORM

Therapist/ Clinic	Address, tel. number	Date
Client's Name	Gender	Doctor's name
Client's address	Age	Doctor's address
Tel. number	Occupation	Doctor's tel. number

GENERAL HEALTH

Symptoms presented by the client for treatment (if any)	General Health

LIFESTYLE/ BACKGROUND INFORMATION

Occupation	Stress level (1-10):	Diet:	Eating patterns
Family circumstances	Exercise	Fluid intake	Sleeping patterns
Relaxation	Alcohol intake	Smoker/non-smoker	Bowels

MEDICAL HISTORY

PAST MEDICAL HISTORY	PRESENT HEALTH
Recent operations	Medical conditions
Serious illnesses, accidents, injuries	Medication taken
Past treatments (received from other therapists or medical ones). When and why?	Current treatments

CONTRA-INDICATIONS/ CAUTIONS

Diabetes/Epilepsy	Arthritis / Rheumatism	Back / Neck Problems
Contagious/Infectious diseases	Moles (large, irregular), warts, skin tags	Cuts / bruises / swellings/recent scars
Heart / Lung disorders	Varicose veins	Undiagnosed lumps /bumps
Cancer	Sunburn/Windburn	Recent hemorrhage
Pregnancy	Allergies, Asthma	Metal pins/plates
Thrombosis / Embolism	Skin disorders / diseases /active shingles	Swollen, hot or painful joints
Fractures / Sprains	Nerve dysfunction (e.g. MS)	Blood pressure disorders

ANY OTHER ISSUES THAT CONCERN YOU

OBJECTIVES OF THE TREATMENT & TREATMENT PLAN

What does the client hope to achieve?	
What will be possible to achieve realistically?	
Treatment plan agreed with the client (number of treatments to be given, over what period of time, length of time between treatments).	

PHYSICAL CONDITION OF THE CLIENT

Observations of the body during treatment (body type; condition of the skin, undiagnosed lumps/bumps, moles, varicose veins, scars, etc.)	
Initial findings after the session (did the client fully relax, was he/she talkative, nervous, any unusual observations, changes?)	

DISCLAIMER

I declare, that all the information regarding me in this form is true and accurate, and as far as I am aware, I can undertake a massage treatment without any adverse effects. I have been fully informed of any contra-indications and I am willing to undertake the treatment with this therapist.

Client's signature...Date...

AFTERCARE ADVICE

CLIENT FEEDBACK/ COMMENTS

Signature .... Date...

REFLEX POINTS – OBSERVATION NOTES

Image credit: https://vecteezy.com

REFLEXOLOGY CONSULTATION FORM

Therapist/ Clinic	Address, tel. number	Date
Client's Name	Gender	Doctor's name
Client's address	Age	Doctor's address
Tel. number	Occupation	Doctor's tel. number

GENERAL HEALTH

Symptoms presented by the client for treatment (if any)	General Health

LIFESTYLE/ BACKGROUND INFORMATION

Occupation	Stress level (1-10):	Diet:	Eating patterns
Family circumstances	Exercise	Fluid intake	Sleeping patterns
Relaxation	Alcohol intake	Smoker/non-smoker	Bowels

MEDICAL HISTORY

PAST MEDICAL HISTORY	PRESENT HEALTH
Recent operations	Medical conditions
Serious illnesses, accidents, injuries	Medication taken
Past treatments (received from other therapists or medical ones). When and why?	Current treatments

CONTRA-INDICATIONS/ CAUTIONS

Diabetes/Epilepsy	Arthritis / Rheumatism	Back / Neck Problems
Contagious/Infectious diseases	Moles (large, irregular), warts, skin tags	Cuts / bruises / swellings/recent scars
Heart / Lung disorders	Varicose veins	Undiagnosed lumps /bumps
Cancer	Sunburn/Windburn	Recent hemorrhage
Pregnancy	Allergies, Asthma	Metal pins/plates
Thrombosis / Embolism	Skin disorders / diseases /active shingles	Swollen, hot or painful joints
Fractures / Sprains	Nerve dysfunction (e.g. MS)	Blood pressure disorders

ANY OTHER ISSUES THAT CONCERN YOU

OBJECTIVES OF THE TREATMENT & TREATMENT PLAN

What does the client hope to achieve?	
What will be possible to achieve realistically?	
Treatment plan agreed with the client (number of treatments to be given, over what period of time, length of time between treatments).	

PHYSICAL CONDITION OF THE CLIENT

Observations of the body during treatment (body type; condition of the skin, undiagnosed lumps/bumps, moles, varicose veins, scars, etc.)	
Initial findings after the session (did the client fully relax, was he/she talkative, nervous, any unusual observations, changes?)	

DISCLAIMER

I declare, that all the information regarding me in this form is true and accurate, and as far as I am aware, I can undertake a massage treatment without any adverse effects. I have been fully informed of any contra-indications and I am willing to undertake the treatment with this therapist.

Client's signature..Date...

AFTERCARE ADVICE

CLIENT FEEDBACK/ COMMENTS

Signature .... Date...

REFLEX POINTS – OBSERVATION NOTES
Image credit: https://vecteezy.com

REFLEXOLOGY CONSULTATION FORM

Therapist/ Clinic	Address, tel. number	Date
Client's Name	Gender	Doctor's name
Client's address	Age	Doctor's address
Tel. number	Occupation	Doctor's tel. number

GENERAL HEALTH

Symptoms presented by the client for treatment (if any)	General Health

LIFESTYLE/ BACKGROUND INFORMATION

Occupation	Stress level (1-10):	Diet:	Eating patterns
Family circumstances	Exercise	Fluid intake	Sleeping patterns
Relaxation	Alcohol intake	Smoker/non-smoker	Bowels

MEDICAL HISTORY

PAST MEDICAL HISTORY	PRESENT HEALTH
Recent operations	Medical conditions
Serious illnesses, accidents, injuries	Medication taken
Past treatments (received from other therapists or medical ones). When and why?	Current treatments

CONTRA-INDICATIONS/ CAUTIONS

Diabetes/Epilepsy	Arthritis / Rheumatism	Back / Neck Problems
Contagious/Infectious diseases	Moles (large, irregular), warts, skin tags	Cuts / bruises / swellings/recent scars
Heart / Lung disorders	Varicose veins	Undiagnosed lumps /bumps
Cancer	Sunburn/Windburn	Recent hemorrhage
Pregnancy	Allergies, Asthma	Metal pins/plates
Thrombosis / Embolism	Skin disorders / diseases /active shingles	Swollen, hot or painful joints
Fractures / Sprains	Nerve dysfunction (e.g. MS)	Blood pressure disorders

ANY OTHER ISSUES THAT CONCERN YOU

OBJECTIVES OF THE TREATMENT & TREATMENT PLAN

What does the client hope to achieve?	
What will be possible to achieve realistically?	
Treatment plan agreed with the client (number of treatments to be given, over what period of time, length of time between treatments).	

PHYSICAL CONDITION OF THE CLIENT

Observations of the body during treatment (body type; condition of the skin, undiagnosed lumps/bumps, moles, varicose veins, scars, etc.)	
Initial findings after the session (did the client fully relax, was he/she talkative, nervous, any unusual observations, changes?)	

DISCLAIMER

I declare, that all the information regarding me in this form is true and accurate, and as far as I am aware, I can undertake a massage treatment without any adverse effects. I have been fully informed of any contra-indications and I am willing to undertake the treatment with this therapist.

Client's signature..Date...

AFTERCARE ADVICE

CLIENT FEEDBACK/ COMMENTS

Signature .... Date...

REFLEX POINTS – OBSERVATION NOTES
Image credit: https://vecteezy.com

REFLEXOLOGY CONSULTATION FORM

Therapist/ Clinic	Address, tel. number	Date
Client's Name	Gender	Doctor's name
Client's address	Age	Doctor's address
Tel. number	Occupation	Doctor's tel. number

GENERAL HEALTH

Symptoms presented by the client for treatment (if any)	General Health

LIFESTYLE/ BACKGROUND INFORMATION

Occupation	Stress level (1-10):	Diet:	Eating patterns
Family circumstances	Exercise	Fluid intake	Sleeping patterns
Relaxation	Alcohol intake	Smoker/non-smoker	Bowels

MEDICAL HISTORY

PAST MEDICAL HISTORY	PRESENT HEALTH
Recent operations	Medical conditions
Serious illnesses, accidents, injuries	Medication taken
Past treatments (received from other therapists or medical ones). When and why?	Current treatments

CONTRA-INDICATIONS/ CAUTIONS

Diabetes/Epilepsy	Arthritis / Rheumatism	Back / Neck Problems
Contagious/Infectious diseases	Moles (large, irregular), warts, skin tags	Cuts / bruises / swellings/recent scars
Heart / Lung disorders	Varicose veins	Undiagnosed lumps /bumps
Cancer	Sunburn/Windburn	Recent hemorrhage
Pregnancy	Allergies, Asthma	Metal pins/plates
Thrombosis / Embolism	Skin disorders / diseases /active shingles	Swollen, hot or painful joints
Fractures / Sprains	Nerve dysfunction (e.g. MS)	Blood pressure disorders

ANY OTHER ISSUES THAT CONCERN YOU

OBJECTIVES OF THE TREATMENT & TREATMENT PLAN

What does the client hope to achieve?	
What will be possible to achieve realistically?	
Treatment plan agreed with the client (number of treatments to be given, over what period of time, length of time between treatments).	

PHYSICAL CONDITION OF THE CLIENT

Observations of the body during treatment (body type; condition of the skin, undiagnosed lumps/bumps, moles, varicose veins, scars, etc.)	
Initial findings after the session (did the client fully relax, was he/she talkative, nervous, any unusual observations, changes?)	

DISCLAIMER

I declare, that all the information regarding me in this form is true and accurate, and as far as I am aware, I can undertake a massage treatment without any adverse effects. I have been fully informed of any contra-indications and I am willing to undertake the treatment with this therapist.

Client's signature...Date..

AFTERCARE ADVICE

CLIENT FEEDBACK/ COMMENTS

Signature .... Date...

REFLEX POINTS – OBSERVATION NOTES
Image credit: https://vecteezy.com

REFLEXOLOGY CONSULTATION FORM

Therapist/ Clinic	Address, tel. number	Date
Client's Name	Gender	Doctor's name
Client's address	Age	Doctor's address
Tel. number	Occupation	Doctor's tel. number

GENERAL HEALTH

Symptoms presented by the client for treatment (if any)	General Health

LIFESTYLE/ BACKGROUND INFORMATION

Occupation	Stress level (1-10):	Diet:	Eating patterns
Family circumstances	Exercise	Fluid intake	Sleeping patterns
Relaxation	Alcohol intake	Smoker/non-smoker	Bowels

MEDICAL HISTORY

PAST MEDICAL HISTORY	PRESENT HEALTH
Recent operations	Medical conditions
Serious illnesses, accidents, injuries	Medication taken
Past treatments (received from other therapists or medical ones). When and why?	Current treatments

CONTRA-INDICATIONS/ CAUTIONS

Diabetes/Epilepsy	Arthritis / Rheumatism	Back / Neck Problems
Contagious/Infectious diseases	Moles (large, irregular), warts, skin tags	Cuts / bruises / swellings/recent scars
Heart / Lung disorders	Varicose veins	Undiagnosed lumps /bumps
Cancer	Sunburn/Windburn	Recent hemorrhage
Pregnancy	Allergies, Asthma	Metal pins/plates
Thrombosis / Embolism	Skin disorders / diseases /active shingles	Swollen, hot or painful joints
Fractures / Sprains	Nerve dysfunction (e.g. MS)	Blood pressure disorders

ANY OTHER ISSUES THAT CONCERN YOU

OBJECTIVES OF THE TREATMENT & TREATMENT PLAN

What does the client hope to achieve?	
What will be possible to achieve realistically?	
Treatment plan agreed with the client (number of treatments to be given, over what period of time, length of time between treatments).	

PHYSICAL CONDITION OF THE CLIENT

Observations of the body during treatment (body type; condition of the skin, undiagnosed lumps/bumps, moles, varicose veins, scars, etc.)	
Initial findings after the session (did the client fully relax, was he/she talkative, nervous, any unusual observations, changes?)	

DISCLAIMER

I declare, that all the information regarding me in this form is true and accurate, and as far as I am aware, I can undertake a massage treatment without any adverse effects. I have been fully informed of any contra-indications and I am willing to undertake the treatment with this therapist.

Client's signature...Date..

AFTERCARE ADVICE

CLIENT FEEDBACK/ COMMENTS

Signature .... Date..

REFLEX POINTS – OBSERVATION NOTES
Image credit: https://vecteezy.com

REFLEXOLOGY CONSULTATION FORM

Therapist/ Clinic	Address, tel. number	Date
Client's Name	Gender	Doctor's name
Client's address	Age	Doctor's address
Tel. number	Occupation	Doctor's tel. number

GENERAL HEALTH

Symptoms presented by the client for treatment (if any)	General Health

LIFESTYLE/ BACKGROUND INFORMATION

Occupation	Stress level (1-10):	Diet:	Eating patterns
Family circumstances	Exercise	Fluid intake	Sleeping patterns
Relaxation	Alcohol intake	Smoker/non-smoker	Bowels

MEDICAL HISTORY

PAST MEDICAL HISTORY	PRESENT HEALTH
Recent operations	Medical conditions
Serious illnesses, accidents, injuries	Medication taken
Past treatments (received from other therapists or medical ones). When and why?	Current treatments

CONTRA-INDICATIONS/ CAUTIONS

Diabetes/Epilepsy	Arthritis / Rheumatism	Back / Neck Problems
Contagious/Infectious diseases	Moles (large, irregular), warts, skin tags	Cuts / bruises / swellings/recent scars
Heart / Lung disorders	Varicose veins	Undiagnosed lumps /bumps
Cancer	Sunburn/Windburn	Recent hemorrhage
Pregnancy	Allergies, Asthma	Metal pins/plates
Thrombosis / Embolism	Skin disorders / diseases /active shingles	Swollen, hot or painful joints
Fractures / Sprains	Nerve dysfunction (e.g. MS)	Blood pressure disorders

ANY OTHER ISSUES THAT CONCERN YOU

OBJECTIVES OF THE TREATMENT & TREATMENT PLAN

What does the client hope to achieve?	
What will be possible to achieve realistically?	
Treatment plan agreed with the client (number of treatments to be given, over what period of time, length of time between treatments).	

PHYSICAL CONDITION OF THE CLIENT

Observations of the body during treatment (body type; condition of the skin, undiagnosed lumps/bumps, moles, varicose veins, scars, etc.)	
Initial findings after the session (did the client fully relax, was he/she talkative, nervous, any unusual observations, changes?)	

DISCLAIMER

I declare, that all the information regarding me in this form is true and accurate, and as far as I am aware, I can undertake a massage treatment without any adverse effects. I have been fully informed of any contra-indications and I am willing to undertake the treatment with this therapist.

Client's signature...Date...

AFTERCARE ADVICE

CLIENT FEEDBACK/ COMMENTS

Signature .... Date...

REFLEX POINTS – OBSERVATION NOTES

Image credit: https://vecteezy.com

REFLEXOLOGY CONSULTATION FORM

Therapist/ Clinic	Address, tel. number	Date
Client's Name	Gender	Doctor's name
Client's address	Age	Doctor's address
Tel. number	Occupation	Doctor's tel. number

GENERAL HEALTH

Symptoms presented by the client for treatment (if any)	General Health

LIFESTYLE/ BACKGROUND INFORMATION

Occupation	Stress level (1-10):	Diet:	Eating patterns
Family circumstances	Exercise	Fluid intake	Sleeping patterns
Relaxation	Alcohol intake	Smoker/non-smoker	Bowels

MEDICAL HISTORY

PAST MEDICAL HISTORY	PRESENT HEALTH
Recent operations	Medical conditions
Serious illnesses, accidents, injuries	Medication taken
Past treatments (received from other therapists or medical ones). When and why?	Current treatments

CONTRA-INDICATIONS/ CAUTIONS

Diabetes/Epilepsy	Arthritis / Rheumatism	Back / Neck Problems
Contagious/Infectious diseases	Moles (large, irregular), warts, skin tags	Cuts / bruises / swellings/recent scars
Heart / Lung disorders	Varicose veins	Undiagnosed lumps /bumps
Cancer	Sunburn/Windburn	Recent hemorrhage
Pregnancy	Allergies, Asthma	Metal pins/plates
Thrombosis / Embolism	Skin disorders / diseases /active shingles	Swollen, hot or painful joints
Fractures / Sprains	Nerve dysfunction (e.g. MS)	Blood pressure disorders

ANY OTHER ISSUES THAT CONCERN YOU

OBJECTIVES OF THE TREATMENT & TREATMENT PLAN

What does the client hope to achieve?	
What will be possible to achieve realistically?	
Treatment plan agreed with the client (number of treatments to be given, over what period of time, length of time between treatments).	

PHYSICAL CONDITION OF THE CLIENT

Observations of the body during treatment (body type; condition of the skin, undiagnosed lumps/bumps, moles, varicose veins, scars, etc.)	
Initial findings after the session (did the client fully relax, was he/she talkative, nervous, any unusual observations, changes?)	

DISCLAIMER

I declare, that all the information regarding me in this form is true and accurate, and as far as I am aware, I can undertake a massage treatment without any adverse effects. I have been fully informed of any contra-indications and I am willing to undertake the treatment with this therapist.

Client's signature...Date..

AFTERCARE ADVICE

CLIENT FEEDBACK/ COMMENTS

Signature .... Date...

REFLEX POINTS – OBSERVATION NOTES
Image credit: https://vecteezy.com

REFLEXOLOGY CONSULTATION FORM

Therapist/ Clinic	Address, tel. number	Date
Client's Name	Gender	Doctor's name
Client's address	Age	Doctor's address
Tel. number	Occupation	Doctor's tel. number

GENERAL HEALTH

Symptoms presented by the client for treatment (if any)	General Health

LIFESTYLE/ BACKGROUND INFORMATION

Occupation	Stress level (1-10):	Diet:	Eating patterns
Family circumstances	Exercise	Fluid intake	Sleeping patterns
Relaxation	Alcohol intake	Smoker/non-smoker	Bowels

MEDICAL HISTORY

PAST MEDICAL HISTORY	PRESENT HEALTH
Recent operations	Medical conditions
Serious illnesses, accidents, injuries	Medication taken
Past treatments (received from other therapists or medical ones). When and why?	Current treatments

CONTRA-INDICATIONS/ CAUTIONS

Diabetes/Epilepsy	Arthritis / Rheumatism	Back / Neck Problems
Contagious/Infectious diseases	Moles (large, irregular), warts, skin tags	Cuts / bruises / swellings/recent scars
Heart / Lung disorders	Varicose veins	Undiagnosed lumps /bumps
Cancer	Sunburn/Windburn	Recent hemorrhage
Pregnancy	Allergies, Asthma	Metal pins/plates
Thrombosis / Embolism	Skin disorders / diseases /active shingles	Swollen, hot or painful joints
Fractures / Sprains	Nerve dysfunction (e.g. MS)	Blood pressure disorders

ANY OTHER ISSUES THAT CONCERN YOU

OBJECTIVES OF THE TREATMENT & TREATMENT PLAN

What does the client hope to achieve?	
What will be possible to achieve realistically?	
Treatment plan agreed with the client (number of treatments to be given, over what period of time, length of time between treatments).	

PHYSICAL CONDITION OF THE CLIENT

Observations of the body during treatment (body type; condition of the skin, undiagnosed lumps/bumps, moles, varicose veins, scars, etc.)	
Initial findings after the session (did the client fully relax, was he/she talkative, nervous, any unusual observations, changes?)	

DISCLAIMER

I declare, that all the information regarding me in this form is true and accurate, and as far as I am aware, I can undertake a massage treatment without any adverse effects. I have been fully informed of any contra-indications and I am willing to undertake the treatment with this therapist.

Client's signature...Date..

AFTERCARE ADVICE

CLIENT FEEDBACK/ COMMENTS

Signature .... Date..

REFLEX POINTS – OBSERVATION NOTES
Image credit: https://vecteezy.com

REFLEXOLOGY CONSULTATION FORM

Therapist/ Clinic	Address, tel. number	Date
Client's Name	Gender	Doctor's name
Client's address	Age	Doctor's address
Tel. number	Occupation	Doctor's tel. number

GENERAL HEALTH

Symptoms presented by the client for treatment (if any)	General Health

LIFESTYLE/ BACKGROUND INFORMATION

Occupation	Stress level (1-10):	Diet:	Eating patterns
Family circumstances	Exercise	Fluid intake	Sleeping patterns
Relaxation	Alcohol intake	Smoker/non-smoker	Bowels

MEDICAL HISTORY

PAST MEDICAL HISTORY	PRESENT HEALTH
Recent operations	Medical conditions
Serious illnesses, accidents, injuries	Medication taken
Past treatments (received from other therapists or medical ones). When and why?	Current treatments

CONTRA-INDICATIONS/ CAUTIONS

Diabetes/Epilepsy	Arthritis / Rheumatism	Back / Neck Problems
Contagious/Infectious diseases	Moles (large, irregular), warts, skin tags	Cuts / bruises / swellings/recent scars
Heart / Lung disorders	Varicose veins	Undiagnosed lumps /bumps
Cancer	Sunburn/Windburn	Recent hemorrhage
Pregnancy	Allergies, Asthma	Metal pins/plates
Thrombosis / Embolism	Skin disorders / diseases /active shingles	Swollen, hot or painful joints
Fractures / Sprains	Nerve dysfunction (e.g. MS)	Blood pressure disorders

ANY OTHER ISSUES THAT CONCERN YOU

OBJECTIVES OF THE TREATMENT & TREATMENT PLAN

What does the client hope to achieve?	
What will be possible to achieve realistically?	
Treatment plan agreed with the client (number of treatments to be given, over what period of time, length of time between treatments).	

PHYSICAL CONDITION OF THE CLIENT

Observations of the body during treatment (body type; condition of the skin, undiagnosed lumps/bumps, moles, varicose veins, scars, etc.)	
Initial findings after the session (did the client fully relax, was he/she talkative, nervous, any unusual observations, changes?)	

DISCLAIMER

I declare, that all the information regarding me in this form is true and accurate, and as far as I am aware, I can undertake a massage treatment without any adverse effects. I have been fully informed of any contra-indications and I am willing to undertake the treatment with this therapist.

Client's signature...Date..

AFTERCARE ADVICE

CLIENT FEEDBACK/ COMMENTS

Signature .... Date..

REFLEX POINTS – OBSERVATION NOTES
Image credit: https://vecteezy.com

REFLEXOLOGY CONSULTATION FORM

Therapist/ Clinic	Address, tel. number	Date
Client's Name	Gender	Doctor's name
Client's address	Age	Doctor's address
Tel. number	Occupation	Doctor's tel. number

GENERAL HEALTH

Symptoms presented by the client for treatment (if any)	General Health

LIFESTYLE/ BACKGROUND INFORMATION

Occupation	Stress level (1-10):	Diet:	Eating patterns
Family circumstances	Exercise	Fluid intake	Sleeping patterns
Relaxation	Alcohol intake	Smoker/non-smoker	Bowels

MEDICAL HISTORY

PAST MEDICAL HISTORY	PRESENT HEALTH
Recent operations	Medical conditions
Serious illnesses, accidents, injuries	Medication taken
Past treatments (received from other therapists or medical ones). When and why?	Current treatments

CONTRA-INDICATIONS/ CAUTIONS

Diabetes/Epilepsy	Arthritis / Rheumatism	Back / Neck Problems
Contagious/Infectious diseases	Moles (large, irregular), warts, skin tags	Cuts / bruises / swellings/recent scars
Heart / Lung disorders	Varicose veins	Undiagnosed lumps /bumps
Cancer	Sunburn/Windburn	Recent hemorrhage
Pregnancy	Allergies, Asthma	Metal pins/plates
Thrombosis / Embolism	Skin disorders / diseases /active shingles	Swollen, hot or painful joints
Fractures / Sprains	Nerve dysfunction (e.g. MS)	Blood pressure disorders

ANY OTHER ISSUES THAT CONCERN YOU

OBJECTIVES OF THE TREATMENT & TREATMENT PLAN

What does the client hope to achieve?	
What will be possible to achieve realistically?	
Treatment plan agreed with the client (number of treatments to be given, over what period of time, length of time between treatments).	

PHYSICAL CONDITION OF THE CLIENT

Observations of the body during treatment (body type; condition of the skin, undiagnosed lumps/bumps, moles, varicose veins, scars, etc.)	
Initial findings after the session (did the client fully relax, was he/she talkative, nervous, any unusual observations, changes?)	

DISCLAIMER

I declare, that all the information regarding me in this form is true and accurate, and as far as I am aware, I can undertake a massage treatment without any adverse effects. I have been fully informed of any contra-indications and I am willing to undertake the treatment with this therapist.

Client's signature...Date...

AFTERCARE ADVICE

CLIENT FEEDBACK/ COMMENTS

Signature .... Date...

REFLEX POINTS – OBSERVATION NOTES
Image credit: https://vecteezy.com

REFLEXOLOGY CONSULTATION FORM

Therapist/ Clinic	Address, tel. number	Date
Client's Name	Gender	Doctor's name
Client's address	Age	Doctor's address
Tel. number	Occupation	Doctor's tel. number

GENERAL HEALTH

Symptoms presented by the client for treatment (if any)	General Health

LIFESTYLE/ BACKGROUND INFORMATION

Occupation	Stress level (1-10):	Diet:	Eating patterns
Family circumstances	Exercise	Fluid intake	Sleeping patterns
Relaxation	Alcohol intake	Smoker/non-smoker	Bowels

MEDICAL HISTORY

PAST MEDICAL HISTORY	PRESENT HEALTH
Recent operations	Medical conditions
Serious illnesses, accidents, injuries	Medication taken
Past treatments (received from other therapists or medical ones). When and why?	Current treatments

CONTRA-INDICATIONS/ CAUTIONS

Diabetes/Epilepsy	Arthritis / Rheumatism	Back / Neck Problems
Contagious/Infectious diseases	Moles (large, irregular), warts, skin tags	Cuts / bruises / swellings/recent scars
Heart / Lung disorders	Varicose veins	Undiagnosed lumps /bumps
Cancer	Sunburn/Windburn	Recent hemorrhage
Pregnancy	Allergies, Asthma	Metal pins/plates
Thrombosis / Embolism	Skin disorders / diseases /active shingles	Swollen, hot or painful joints
Fractures / Sprains	Nerve dysfunction (e.g. MS)	Blood pressure disorders

ANY OTHER ISSUES THAT CONCERN YOU

OBJECTIVES OF THE TREATMENT & TREATMENT PLAN

What does the client hope to achieve?	
What will be possible to achieve realistically?	
Treatment plan agreed with the client (number of treatments to be given, over what period of time, length of time between treatments).	

PHYSICAL CONDITION OF THE CLIENT

Observations of the body during treatment (body type; condition of the skin, undiagnosed lumps/bumps, moles, varicose veins, scars, etc.)	
Initial findings after the session (did the client fully relax, was he/she talkative, nervous, any unusual observations, changes?)	

DISCLAIMER

I declare, that all the information regarding me in this form is true and accurate, and as far as I am aware, I can undertake a massage treatment without any adverse effects. I have been fully informed of any contra-indications and I am willing to undertake the treatment with this therapist.

Client's signature...Date..

AFTERCARE ADVICE

CLIENT FEEDBACK/ COMMENTS

Signature .... Date..

REFLEX POINTS – OBSERVATION NOTES
Image credit: https://vecteezy.com

REFLEXOLOGY CONSULTATION FORM

Therapist/ Clinic	Address, tel. number	Date
Client's Name	Gender	Doctor's name
Client's address	Age	Doctor's address
Tel. number	Occupation	Doctor's tel. number

GENERAL HEALTH

Symptoms presented by the client for treatment (if any)	General Health

LIFESTYLE/ BACKGROUND INFORMATION

Occupation	Stress level (1-10):	Diet:	Eating patterns
Family circumstances	Exercise	Fluid intake	Sleeping patterns
Relaxation	Alcohol intake	Smoker/non-smoker	Bowels

MEDICAL HISTORY

PAST MEDICAL HISTORY	PRESENT HEALTH
Recent operations	Medical conditions
Serious illnesses, accidents, injuries	Medication taken
Past treatments (received from other therapists or medical ones). When and why?	Current treatments

CONTRA-INDICATIONS/ CAUTIONS

Diabetes/Epilepsy	Arthritis / Rheumatism	Back / Neck Problems
Contagious/Infectious diseases	Moles (large, irregular), warts, skin tags	Cuts / bruises / swellings/recent scars
Heart / Lung disorders	Varicose veins	Undiagnosed lumps /bumps
Cancer	Sunburn/Windburn	Recent hemorrhage
Pregnancy	Allergies, Asthma	Metal pins/plates
Thrombosis / Embolism	Skin disorders / diseases /active shingles	Swollen, hot or painful joints
Fractures / Sprains	Nerve dysfunction (e.g. MS)	Blood pressure disorders

ANY OTHER ISSUES THAT CONCERN YOU

OBJECTIVES OF THE TREATMENT & TREATMENT PLAN

What does the client hope to achieve?	
What will be possible to achieve realistically?	
Treatment plan agreed with the client (number of treatments to be given, over what period of time, length of time between treatments).	

PHYSICAL CONDITION OF THE CLIENT

Observations of the body during treatment (body type; condition of the skin, undiagnosed lumps/bumps, moles, varicose veins, scars, etc.)	
Initial findings after the session (did the client fully relax, was he/she talkative, nervous, any unusual observations, changes?)	

DISCLAIMER

I declare, that all the information regarding me in this form is true and accurate, and as far as I am aware, I can undertake a massage treatment without any adverse effects. I have been fully informed of any contra-indications and I am willing to undertake the treatment with this therapist.

Client's signature...Date...

AFTERCARE ADVICE

CLIENT FEEDBACK/ COMMENTS

Signature .... Date...

REFLEX POINTS – OBSERVATION NOTES

Image credit: https://vecteezy.com

REFLEXOLOGY CONSULTATION FORM

Therapist/ Clinic	Address, tel. number	Date
Client's Name	Gender	Doctor's name
Client's address	Age	Doctor's address
Tel. number	Occupation	Doctor's tel. number

GENERAL HEALTH

Symptoms presented by the client for treatment (if any)	General Health

LIFESTYLE/ BACKGROUND INFORMATION

Occupation	Stress level (1-10):	Diet:	Eating patterns
Family circumstances	Exercise	Fluid intake	Sleeping patterns
Relaxation	Alcohol intake	Smoker/non-smoker	Bowels

MEDICAL HISTORY

PAST MEDICAL HISTORY	PRESENT HEALTH
Recent operations	Medical conditions
Serious illnesses, accidents, injuries	Medication taken
Past treatments (received from other therapists or medical ones). When and why?	Current treatments

CONTRA-INDICATIONS/ CAUTIONS

Diabetes/Epilepsy	Arthritis / Rheumatism	Back / Neck Problems
Contagious/Infectious diseases	Moles (large, irregular), warts, skin tags	Cuts / bruises / swellings/recent scars
Heart / Lung disorders	Varicose veins	Undiagnosed lumps /bumps
Cancer	Sunburn/Windburn	Recent hemorrhage
Pregnancy	Allergies, Asthma	Metal pins/plates
Thrombosis / Embolism	Skin disorders / diseases /active shingles	Swollen, hot or painful joints
Fractures / Sprains	Nerve dysfunction (e.g. MS)	Blood pressure disorders

ANY OTHER ISSUES THAT CONCERN YOU

OBJECTIVES OF THE TREATMENT & TREATMENT PLAN

What does the client hope to achieve?	
What will be possible to achieve realistically?	
Treatment plan agreed with the client (number of treatments to be given, over what period of time, length of time between treatments).	

PHYSICAL CONDITION OF THE CLIENT

Observations of the body during treatment (body type; condition of the skin, undiagnosed lumps/bumps, moles, varicose veins, scars, etc.)	
Initial findings after the session (did the client fully relax, was he/she talkative, nervous, any unusual observations, changes?)	

DISCLAIMER

I declare, that all the information regarding me in this form is true and accurate, and as far as I am aware, I can undertake a massage treatment without any adverse effects. I have been fully informed of any contra-indications and I am willing to undertake the treatment with this therapist.

Client's signature...Date..

AFTERCARE ADVICE

CLIENT FEEDBACK/ COMMENTS

Signature .... Date..

REFLEX POINTS – OBSERVATION NOTES
Image credit: https://vecteezy.com

Appointments

Name	Phone Number	Date/Time	Notes

Appointments

Name	Phone Number	Date/Time	Notes

Appointments

Name	Phone Number	Date/ Time	Notes

Appointments

Name	Phone Number	Date/ Time	Notes

Appointments

Name	Phone Number	Date/ Time	Notes

Appointments

Name	Phone Number	Date/Time	Notes

Appointments

Name	Phone Number	Date/ Time	Notes

Appointments

Name	Phone Number	Date/Time	Notes

Appointments

Name	Phone Number	Date/Time	Notes

Appointments

Name	Phone Number	Date/Time	Notes

Appointments

Name	Phone Number	Date/Time	Notes

Appointments

Name	Phone Number	Date/Time	Notes

Notes

Notes

Notes

Notes

Notes

Notes

Printed in Great Britain
by Amazon

26393819R00071